DOWN THERE

Narratives about the joy, aroma and
overall existence of the bush.

Book design by Georgia Scott. Text set in Lyon Text Short G1.

Library of Congress Cataloging-in-Publication data
Scott, Georgia
Down There / Georgia Scott
ISBN-13: 978-0983207214 (Treadwater Breathe)
ISBN-10: 0983207216
Third Edition

There are two kinds of men. Those who like it shaved and those who don't. But I

think regardless of the type, they are all turned on by the "idea" of a woman shaving. I mean, if a man calls a woman and asks what she's doing, and she says that she's about to shave her lady parts, he's going to react in a certain kind of way. Even if he's the type to not usually care about pubic hair. The imagination is a powerful thing.

I have a long distance relationship and my boyfriend and use Skype to have online sex. I think because of that, the vsual s mch me mportant.

Women:

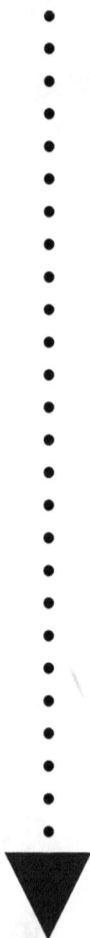

Trimming

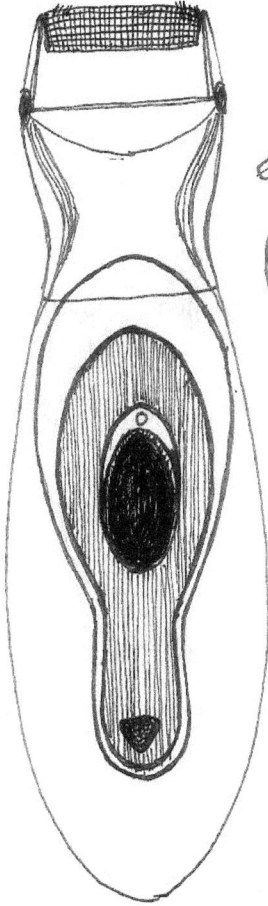

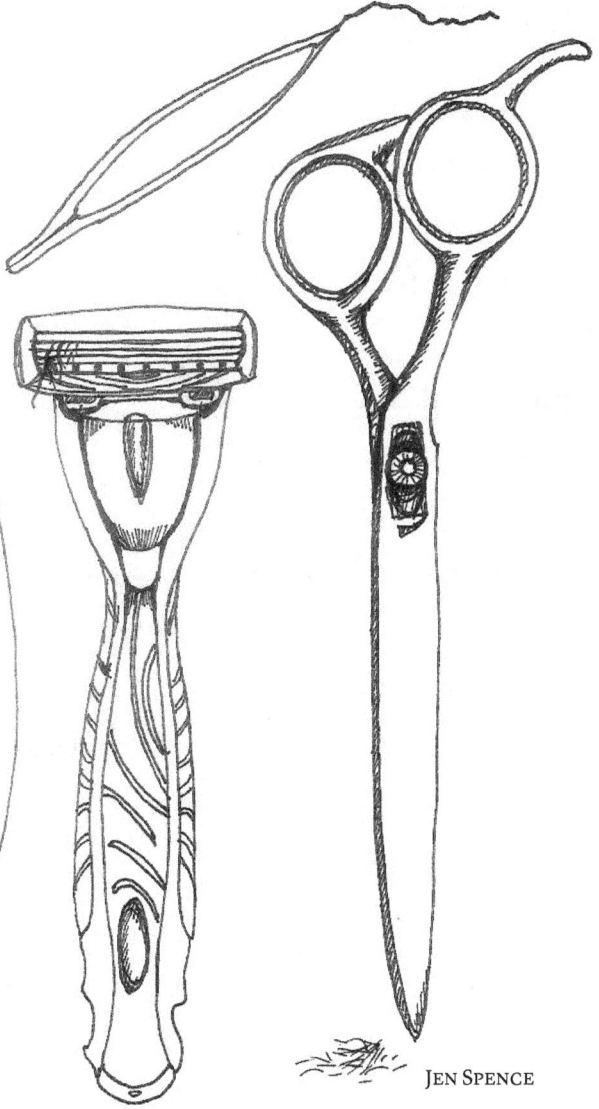

JEN SPENCE

I'm really hairy down there. Really. No, really.

And it's thick from my thighs to my ankles. My doctor asked what did I expect because I have thick hair on my head, so of course it's going to be thick down there.

Fine. But mine is woolly mammoth thick. And my skin is super sensitive, so I can't shave. I trim my pubic hair and the area around my panty line and upper thighs, but I can't go very low. The only parts I can shave are my lower legs, up to about two inches above my knees, which allows me to at least wear long shorts.

I explain clearly to every guy I date, "This is it and this is why. You have to take it or leave it." They've always been fine with it, but then my current boyfriend—and I love him, I really do—said to me, "I've never known anyone that didn't shave their pubic hair." That really hurt. I mean, I was always self-conscious of it, even before he made that comment, but then that made me feel completely awful.

The first time I saw a gray hair, I attempted to pluck it, completely miscalculating how painful it would be.

I thought it would be simple, and that if I yanked it out fast enough, I'd just feel a pinch but that's it. You're laughing, but I'm being serious. I thought it'd be the same like when I see a gray hair on my head. I yank it, no problem. But oh my God! I almost fainted. That was three years ago and I never tried again. It's still there.

I always thought I kept my pubic hair trimmed pretty low, but it's not like I had anyone to compare it to. So when a guy complained that my pubic hair was too long, I thought to myself, "Seriously?!" And then I said out loud, a little pissed off and defensively, "No it's not. I trim."

"Not enough," he said. To which I replied, "Damn, how much more can I cut off?"

"A lot," he said.

He ghosted me after that. I think about that night every time I trim, and make a conscious effort to get extremely low. I feel like my pubic hair was this arbitrary reason I lost a really good guy. I don't want that to ever happen again.

I was in my 20s when I decided I should at least trim for bathing suits. Back then, I

thought it was enough to shave around the bikini line. But I didn't think about trimming the actual bush. Then in my 30s, I decided to get waxed before a vacation—going from zero to everything on a whim. Now in my 40s, I've been experimenting a bit more. My favorite is the Brazilian with a thin landing strip. The first time I saw it was weird, and different and crazy. I thought it was very European.

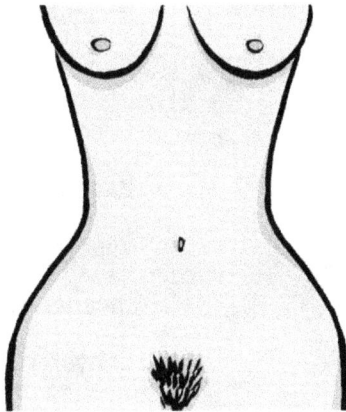

Veronica Malatesta

I don't like a lot of pubic hair

and generally keep it pretty trimmed. But when I'm in a relationship, I make more of an effort to keep it tight. I mean meticulously groomed so he won't have NO problems finding what he needs to find. It's right there and it's sticking out. No excuses.

Even though I like how everything looks

when it's trimmed, it seems like there's always something else more pressing to do. But then when I finally get around to it, I get disgusted at how long the hair has grown. To make matters worse, right before I begin, I always have to pee. Then urine gets on the hair and no matter how much I wipe, my bush stays wet. Which means now I have to trim a lot of overgrown, pissy-damp hair. So gross!

I've heard so many horror stories about men making cruel comments about a woman's bush. Thank God the first comment about my foliage was a compliment. I went home one night with a bouncer at a nightclub in NYC. We smoked up a bit, kissed a bit, and when I took off my underwear, he had this incredible reaction. I was laying on his bed and he just started playing with my pubic hair with his hands and lips, like he was tugging at it and rubbing on it. He told me he was so used to everyone shaving, that he'd forgotten what it was like to see so much "bush." I think that was the first time I heard it called that. He also called it an afro. I was a little embarrassed, but he seemed so excited that it made me feel comfortable. He just wanted to play with it for a while.

I like to keep a strip. I feel like sex is better that way. I feel more of everything when I don't have any hair. Getting it waxed really hurts. I ain't gon' lie. But it gets easier. After each waxing, I touch it up myself with a razor.

I was trimming one night before a big date, and I nicked my clit. I was in a rush, which was my first mistake. The second was that I was too focused on the base of the scissors and didn't think about the tip. I screammed. I screamed! I fuckin' screamed so loud! Not because it hurt— although hell yeah, it hurt. But because I immediately knew I'd have to cancel my date.

I grew up in Catholic school and didn't have a lot of exposure to other women,

so I never had any reason to think that there was something unique going on between our legs. One of my friends in the neighborhood asked me once, "You've never ever seen anybody naked?"

No. Not even my mom. Everything was filtered and repressed. My first awareness of pubic hair was on a nude beach in Los Angeles, called Pirate's Cove. There was a huge culture of nudists. They invited me, and I think I was curious to see what it was like. This was decades ago. People weren't shaving everything back then.

That's when I first realized what pubic hair was and that everyone has something different. Mine is dark, some were light. Some were bushier or longer than others. At first, it was hard not to stare.

I started trimming and edging when I was a teenager. I asked my mum what she thought about it. I was afraid she'd be angry, like I'd done something wrong. But she wasn't. She just said it's not something we do and that I've always been different. We're Shona from Zimbabwe and I guess she was talking about all Shona women, or maybe just our family. We never talked about it again.

Women are posting photos of their bush on the internet. And they don't mind showing their faces either. And the thing is, it's not gross or weird. Okay, it's a little weird, but only because it's so unusual. But when you think about it, it's kind of cool. I don't have a full-length mirror so I only see mine when I look down. It's kind of informative to see it straight on from the front, especially when it's in a way that's not sexualized.

For the longest time, my pube was wild and hairy. My mother never talked about anything remotely concerning the va-jay-jay, and I just figured it was supposed to be like that. Then, in my 30s, I dated someone from California. He went down on me, came up, and told me he'd gotten hair in his mouth. He didn't say it in a joking, as-a-matter-of-fact kind of way, but as a complaint. I didn't understand why he was so mad or what he wanted me to say. Later, he said, "You should trim that," with an emphasis on "that" like it was an alien or a curse.

In the German town where I used to work in as an au pair, women never groomed. At all. They seriously think men like all of that hair. One of my neighbors who was always at the pool had a giant bush that spread out like weeds from her bikini, like it wanted to say hello to everyone. It was so thick, it looked like someone had stuffed a small creature down there. You half expected it to start moving.

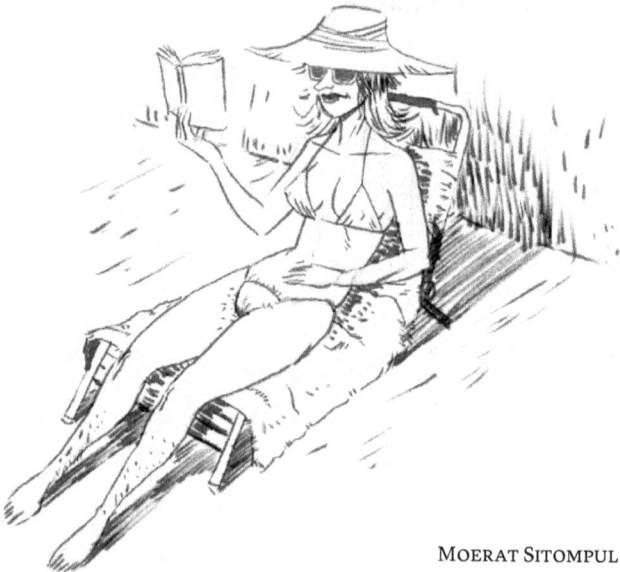

Moerat Sitompul

What do you call your vagina?

PRECIOUS LADY

Cyat

Cat

Cunt

POOTANG

Twat

Pussy

Yoni

Muschi

Moo-Moo

PEACH

Your Breakfast

PLUM Muffin

Hooha

Coochie

NAPPY DUGOUT

Honkey Hideout

HAPPY TRAIL

Poom-Poom

Pandora's Box

LANDING STRIP

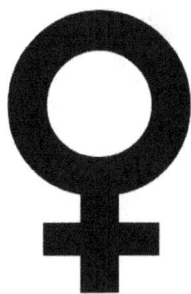

Women:

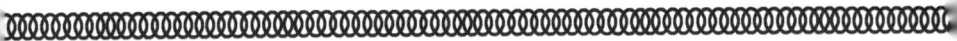

Total removal

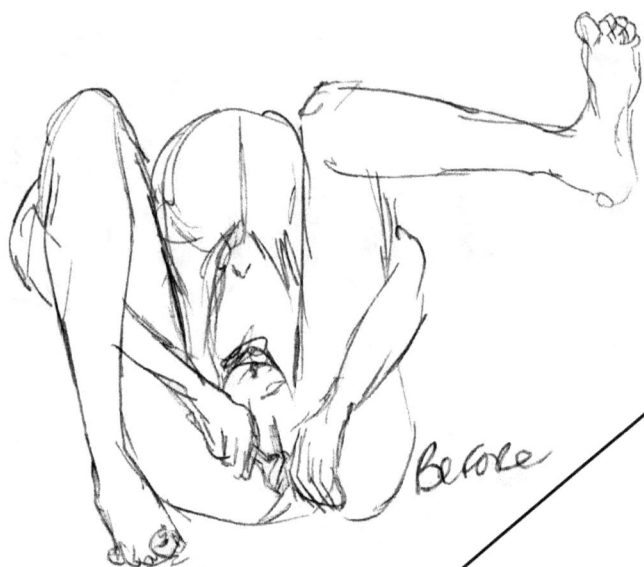

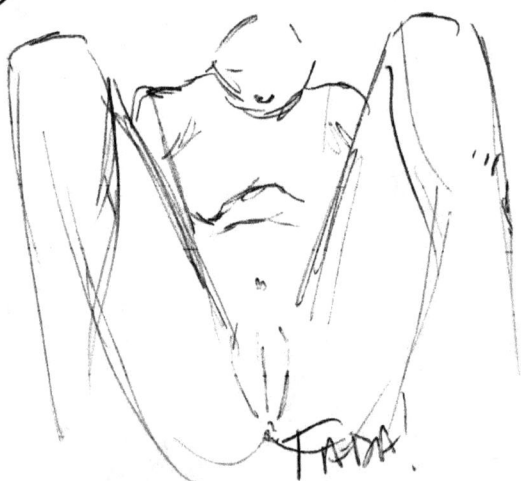

Before

TADA!

AFTER

JEN SPENCE

After I wax, my pubic hair grows back soft, which is nice because I'm very hairy and it's normally coarse and thick. I've heard the horror stories, so I feel pretty lucky. My secret is loofah. I use hot water and loofah it up. It takes off that dead skin layer and keeps the skin fresh.

I invest in a really good, natural loofah, not those plastic scrunchies. That area is tender, so I wet the loofah and gently buff the area. You can't scrub it rough like you do your legs.

My husband thinks that all of this talk about going completely bare is bullshit. I don't agree that it's bullshit, but I love that he loves me just the way I am.

My boyfriend surprised me one day by suggesting we shave our pubic hair together.

I was nervous at first, but he was really sweet and gentle the whole time. He sat me down on the edge of the bathtub and showed me what to do. We'd been dating for years so he's seen me naked hundreds of times. Thousands. But this felt different. I can't explain it. He watched me as I shaved it off. Then I watched as he shaved. Then we rubbed oil on each other and ... Everything was really nice.

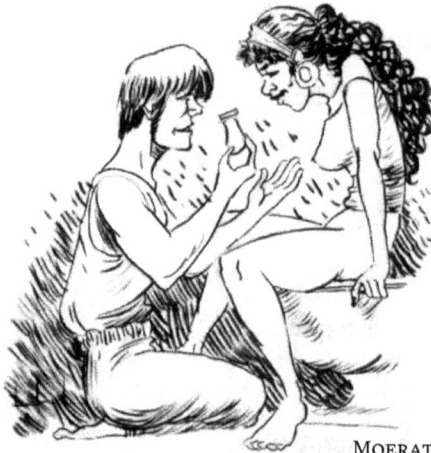

MOERAT SITOMPUL

My roommate and I made a pact to wax

together. I bought two home waxing kits, one for each of us.
She'd never been interested in that sort of thing, but I really wanted
to do it, and didn't want to do it by myself.

The whole thing was an epic fail. First of all, the instructions
were unbelievably vague. Which was made even worse because she's
terrible at reading instuctions. There I was, lying down on a towel on
the living room floor with no underwear on, and my bottom beauty
in her hands. She melted the wax just fine but then she spread way
too much onto my crotch AND my skin. And she hadn't read how to
remove it. She started to panic. I had to take the box from her, read
the instructions myself, then explain them to her. It took so long that
the wax cooled solid. It was impossible to rip it off without taking my
skin with it.

It took over an hour to handle it. On the parts where it stuck to
my pubic hair, we slowly cut off the wax little by little. But the part
where it was stuck to my skin!!! I almost fainted from the pain.

I hate (hate!) having pubic hair.

What's the purpose? It makes everything extra sweaty. I know it's meant to keep stuff out, but it gets on my freaking nerves and makes me smell like a fucking pig. At first I was worried what a guy would think if I took it all off but then I was like, "Fuck him!" I decided I really didn't care. Shaving it completely off is more comfortable for me.

When you get a Brazilian, your leg is hiked up and

the technician is groping at hair everywhere. It took a minute for me to be ok with that.

You're talking about trimming and manicuring the horticulture, right?

I started shaving 15 years ago when I first saw a gray hair. Before that, I was big into NOT shaving. Nothing: not the pits, my legs, the garden—as I like to call it—nothing. I wasn't grooming at all. It didn't go with my personality. I liked being natural. I had a nice little afro under each arm, and a nice hedge in the garden.

Then I saw my first gray hair down there. I went out and bought a Wahl peanut clipper—the cutest little buzz cut razor—and shaved it all off. OMG! It totally increases your sexual satisfaction. The first time I had sex after shaving, I was on the ceiling. I mean, I was typically on the ceiling anyway, but this was off the charts—Cathedral style!

I don't have a lot of body hair, but I have a lot of pubic hair. At that time it was long

enough to braid. My friends were waxing and shaving and I think it just kinda crept into the back of my mind. I'd been dating my boyfriend for about two years. When I mentioned it to him, I thought he'd just agree or disagree, but he surprised me and said let's just try it. "LET'S!" He wanted to be an active participant. The next thing I knew, he had laid a towel on the bed and I was taking my clothes off. He used scissors to cut my bush low, then he lathered it up. It was really intimate. And I feel like it actually brought us closer together.

I think my ex is seeing someone because she started shaving.

She never shaved when we were together. We had always trimmed the bikini line, but never cared about the rest. Last year, we spent Christmas together. I saw that she was completely shaved, which makes me think she's dating someone new and is now concerned about that part of her appearance. Hmmm.

The first time I shaved, I was still in high school. I was

trying to be more feminine. I thought being feminine meant removing as much hair as possible. At the time, I had underarm hair, sideburns, everything. I didn't feel normal. I didn't feel feminine. Looking back, I honestly didn't know how to be feminine and thought shaving was the answer. I couldn't talk to my father or stepmother about it. Instead, I just went overboard and got rid of all of it.

I pluck my pubic hair with tweezers. Each

and every strand, individually. It's what works best for me. I don't
have the money for waxing or expensive depilatories, and my skin is
too sensitive for razors. It hurt a lot at first, but I'm used to it. I barely
feel it now. I just relax, pour myself a glass of wine, and take my time.
I usually do it in intervals—a little bit here and there when I'm at
home. I've been doing it so long that there are patches where the hair
doesn't even grow anymore.

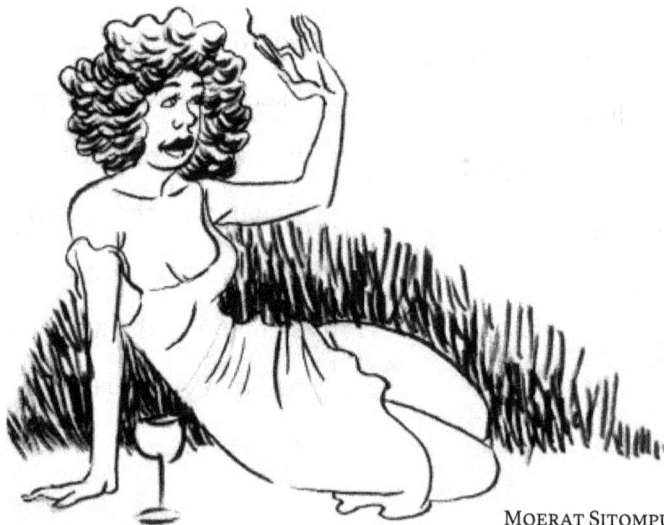

MOERAT SITOMPUL

I'm sure the woman at the spa knows I'm not having sex because

when I am, I see her every two or three weeks to wax it off. So when I don't show up for a while, she knows I'm bushy and back to being single.

The first time I went to a waxing salon, the receptionist made me feel horrible.

I told her I'd never been waxed before and that I was a little scared. She said, "Oh honey, everybody does it," like I'm a child. It took so much courage to make the decision to go. I had never really talked to anybody about it, and so when she said that, I thought wow, I am so late on this.

When I first fully removed my pubic hair, I was in high school. I used Nair which got it baby-booty clean. I mean it was smooth and shiny. But when it started to grow back... omg, the itch! I didn't know about re-growth. All I knew was that my coochie was on fire! I was like, "Why is my coochie on fire?!!" Whenever I walked, I had to hold my jeans away from my body. People thought I looked crazy so I was screaming, "I can't walk cause my coochie's lit up!"

The one & only time I shaved it all off was a few years after I got married. We were going on vacation and I imagined that it would be this amazing, heightened experience. But it was awful. My husband still had all of his hair, so there was so much friction! I had nothing to protect me. The sex—the moving back and forth—was so scratchy and uncomfortable.

Oh my God, let me tell you! The one and only time

I got a full Brazilian wax, it looked cute for a while, but when that shit started to grow back, it was nothing nice. I got ingrown hair bumps from my coochie to my knees. I was in agony. My ass and my coochie felt like a battle zone!

Why my ass? Cause those freaks at the waxing salon got the hair up in the crack too! There was nothing I could do for a week until the hair grew back. It was war!

The first time I shaved was the night before a major surgery.

I wanted to shave it myself instead of the doctors. Then I went to the hospital and realized that none of that was necessary. I had done it all for nothing. But as it turns out, I liked it and now I shave all the time.

People tell you stories about their pubic hair? What?! I'm dumbfounded.

(a few minutes later...)

Actually, my pubic hair started growing when I was in elementary school. So it was always just a natural part of me. I was taught to shave under my arms but there was never any mention about down there. Then in my 20s, after I had my twins, I wanted to experiment. First trimming, then shaving. The shaving, itself, was fine. But it grew back really fast and it was pokey, you know what I mean? And it took a long time to grow out of that pokey stage. I had to scratch a lot. It was kinda embarrassing—scratching my coochie. After that, I just felt like it wasn't worth it to ever do again.

I'm 52 years old, which in my opinion is too old to be shaving for aesthetics.

But being older means my bladder has gotten weaker. I find that I can't hold my pee as long as I used to. One minute I feel like I've got time to finish what I'm doing, and then the next, I'm rushing to the bathroom damn near about to piss myself. When that happens, if I don't keep it waxed, the hair around my panty line gets caught in the elastic. The women at the gym just think I'm being hip. But the reason is much more practical.

For years, I just shaved my underarms and legs. But as I got older, I realized the aesthetics required I start trimming my pubic hair. Then at some point, I went full on. I waxed the lips, the crack, everything. I thought the area around the lips would hurt, but it didn't. It is a little uncomfortable every time, but I only go to one person. She knows me and I trust her.

After the women at the wax salon rip off your hair, I don't get why they want to take the wax strip and show you. It's so nasty. I don't want to see that.

The first time I tried to wax myself, I was bleeding.

Some people think it's enough to only shave the straggling hairs around the bikini line. But when you're skipping around on the beach, playing in the water, wiping sand off with your towel, sitting down with your legs spread open—you DO know that the bikini shifts? And all of that stuff you were too lazy to shave, we see. And it looks nasty.

VERONICA MALATESTA

Personally, I like sugaring because I am very, very afraid of cutting myself.

I think I'd die if I accidentally cut myself. I heard that women in the Middle East do sugaring, especially before they get married. The ancient Egyptians did it as well. I did a lot of research for alternatives to using a razor. Rubbing a homemade concoction of lime juice and sugar over my body seemed a lot more practical. I started with my legs and underarms, and then my eyebrows. (That didn't work out so well.) The first time I used it on my vagina was amazing. It's less irritation, and I never get ingrown hairs.

In Islamic theology, removing unwanted hair from the body is an act of fitrah, which encompasses circumcision, shaving pubic hair, plucking out armpit hair, clipping the nails and trimming facial hair; and that a woman is obligated to shave if her husband orders her to do so. Most Imams say we can remove our pubic hair with anything we prefer, but because a blade is specifically referred to in the teachings, that shaving is the best method.

This isn't like me, but actually right now,

I'm wearing these knee-high socks because I didn't shave my legs. And if I didn't shave my legs, you know what else I didn't shave.

I have long hairs in my butt, so I

have to shave. When they get too long, they tickle. And then I want to scratch. Especially when I'm at work. But I can't do that because then I'll have to go wash my hands. So for me, it's easier to shave everything off.

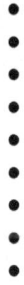

Women:

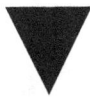

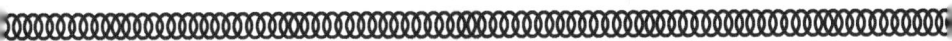

What men say

I like it shaved. I love when the lips are clean. They seem juicier. I don't mind when

there's a small bush. I just don't like it when it's too bushy. But still when the lips are shaved—mmmm, it's just good like that.

I think all women should at least trim. It makes better sex, and I'm aiming for orgasm. When it's not trimmed, it can be a turn off. Like if I go down there and it's a jungle, I'm not going to stay. I'll still do it because I like pussy. But I don't like it as much with a lot of bush, and I'm not going to stay down there for a long time. I'll stay for as long as I can and hopefully it's enough to get the orgasm, but then I'm coming up. Eating pussy is my art, and I want to enjoy it.

My girl only shaves in the summer when it's time to wear shorts and swimsuits.

When she does, there are certain things she's more willing to do sexually. Things she won't do when she has pubic hair. So, the winter months can get kind of long. We've talked about it, but she won't budge. She says that's her break time and that her vagina needs the hair to keep warm. That sounds like bullshit, but what can I do?

I have a whorish disposition regarding size, shape, hair and no hair, in that I'm sort of a "cliché, rugged, equal opportunity, whatever-you-got-bring-it on" kind of guy. Put another way, there's a sermon called "Just As I Am" by Billy Graham with a remarkable message: "Whoever I am, God not only accepts me but He wants me." To borrow from that ideology, if I'm attracted to someone sexually there's nothing about that part of the body that is going to affect me so much that I'm going to change my mind—whether it's bushy enough to be called a jungle, or so shaven it's like a polished jewel. It's very difficult to turn me off once I'm turned on.

Women "deal break" in the moment. Men deal break in the process.

In my mind, I'm not even trying to break deals. I'm just trying to move through the labyrinth. Pubic hair is not my issue. I don't find it attractive nor unattractive. I don't judge. I'm sort of a feel-people-out kind of guy. If we get to that point, then I want to be there. I want to be there in a major way.

Why would I want it completely shaven?

I saw that on my little niece and I'm not about to start sexualizing that. It was really hard to stay in a sexual moment the first time I saw a woman clean-shaven. I don't know what to tell you. It's just really hard to sexualize a vagina that looks like a child's.

I think this whole craze is just a phenomenon. It's porn culture, and that's not where I'm at.

As you take me down my bush memory lane, there was one woman I loved who had a real tight, tight afro. The curls were like a shield of armor. My goodness, it was beautiful.

I've thought about this over the years. When I was younger, no one really trimmed the bush. All the women—black and white—had afros between their thighs. Now as of late, my 40-year-old wife is practically bald down there. I don't know if that's capturing her youth, or if she's trying to hide the gray. I also don't know if I like it.

I don't like the super-duper fros, but I find bush to be a bit intriguing. That's

how I got together with my friend's ex-girlfriend. He had been complaining about how much hair she had. I told him to ask her about it. But his way of asking was to show up one night with clippers. He handled it completely wrong and they broke up.

She asked me what I thought about it. I told her that in general, I don't have a problem with it, but that I'd have to see it to offer an opinion. She invited me over. I know it sounds like I backstabbed my friend, but everything just played out organically. We had drinks. She took off her clothes. I told her she was beautiful and that my friend was an idiot. We started dating after that. She was everything and I should have married her.

I think women shave too much.

On the night of my honeymoon my new wife—my beautiful bride—showed up with all of her pubic hair shaved off. It was supposed to be her gift to me. We'd dated for six years and in all that time, she had barely ever trimmed. Now she was as smooth as a..., I don't even want to think about it. What she thought would be sexy, actually made me uncomfortable.

I didn't say anything, but after we returned from the honeymoon, she kept doing it. I finally had to tell her I wasn't turned on by that. I didn't like seeing a raw, naked vagina.

When I first started eating pussy, hair really didn't matter. And that first girl I was with...

woooh! Her shit wasn't shaved at all, but nobody was doing that back then. If someone was shaving, I didn't know about it.

Maybe that was one reason a lot of men didn't eat out. Cause their women didn't shave. I always thought it was more of a myth, rather than something real people actually did. I remember the first time I saw a woman with her pubic hair completely shaved. I was shocked. I was turned on, I can't lie. Yes, I was. It was a beautiful thing to look at.

It's like the grass in my front yard.

I like a nice lawn. I like when women take care of themselves and at least keep the sides of the triangle trim.

This might be going too far, but there's a pretty pussy, and an ugly one.

The hair needs to be trimmed so I can see which one she has. I also like it trimmed enough so I can see if she's got an outie or an innie. You know, some women have lips that are "out" and some have more of a slit. I've had it both ways. I can't say I have a preference. I just like knowing.

No one wants to be down there licking something that's a mess.

My experiences with women and sexuality are overwhelmingly positive. With regard to the bush, I give it 99% thumbs up.

Hygiene:

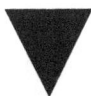

From men and women

Men and women get caught up about the wrong stuff. Shave or don't shave; boxers or briefs; lace or cotton. None of that is as important as good, basic hygiene. If you can maintain that, you've got my attention.

I used to go jogging as far as I could—I'd run until I got tired and couldn't run anymore. Then I would take my time wandering back home. Meandering here and there, eating street food and soaking up the vitamin D. I thought I was being really healthy, not realizing that I was creating an ecosystem of bacteria down there. Now I carry a change of underwear in my fanny pack.

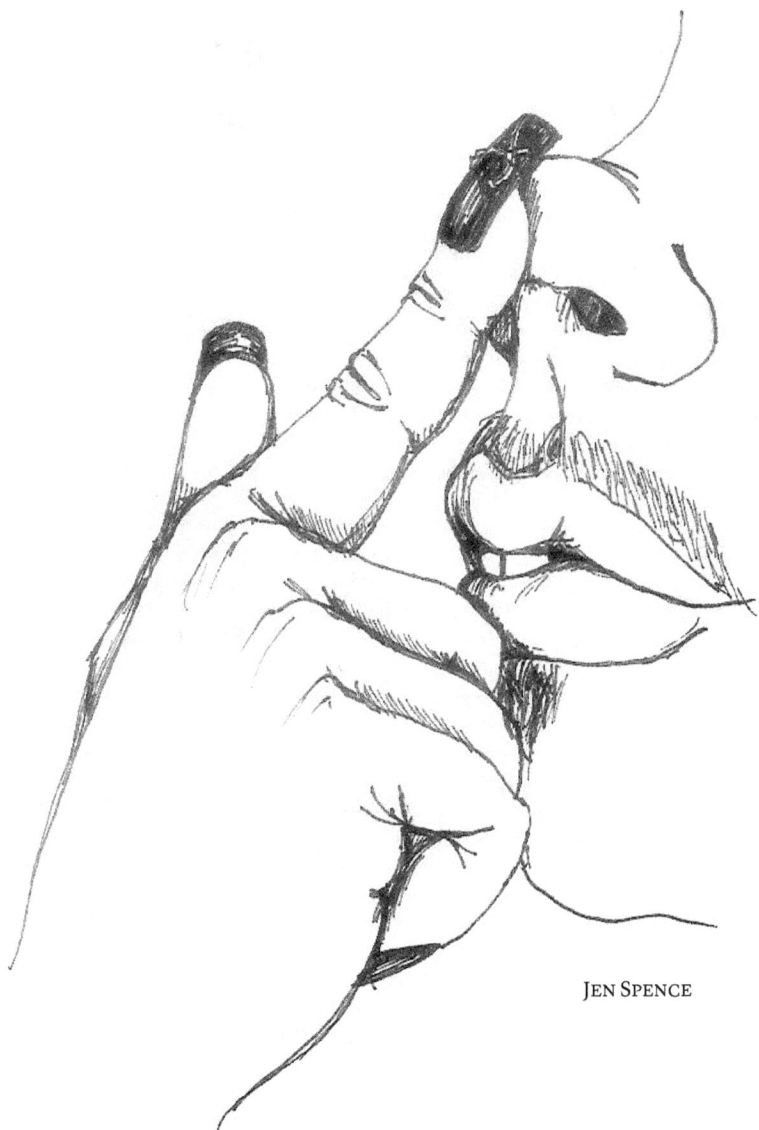

JEN SPENCE

Men and women should always wash their own underwear. I tell my children the same thing my mother told me. "Wash your underwear separately so the smell doesn't get on your clothes. And never rely on other people to wash your underwear." I don't care if they're married. Some things should be kept secret.

When I was in college, the career placement department had a checklist for personal hygiene. It talked about doing this and that—like brushing your teeth and ironing your clothes—before going on a job interview. I think that wisdom extends to any situation, most especially dating. How can you expect to find someone who respects you and loves you if you don't love and respect yourself enough to maintain good hygiene?

When it comes to hygiene, the one thing I find most disgusting is when women try on swimsuits without their panties on. One, you don't know whose crotch was in that bikini before yours. And two, the person behind you doesn't want your smelly cooties.

I shave now but before, I was looking like Willie Nelson. During that era, I was dating a colleague from work. We had sex at the job one day and I didn't get a chance to shower first. I know it must have been smelly, and I feel like the odor lingered in the office. I also wasn't able to wash up afterward, so I remember that day as kind of a low point in my self respect.

Douching is a very American thing.

I moved to the States when I was 16 and some of the other girls were talking about it after volleyball practice. I asked my mom about it and she told me not to. But the other girls made me feel dirty, like I didn't care about hygiene. So I ignored my mom and caved in to peer pressure. That's how I started douching.

I heard douching was bad for you, so I never got into it. I think I might have done it twice in my lifetime.

I moved to Naples with my Italian boyfriend and, you know, Italians are obsessed with cleanliness and everyone has a bidet. It was my first time seeing one and I asked him what it's for. He explained the basics, but as I made friends and asked about the culture of it, they all laughed at me. Everyone uses it after taking a poop. And women especially use it before going to bed. It gives a nice crisp, fresh feeling. We don't use regular shower soap. The markets sell rows of intimate soap that's more delicate for down there.

When a tumor started growing in my head, it changed the way my body smells.

Before that, I'd never thought about shaving. But when it became a matter of hygiene, I had to stop going *au naturel.*

You don't have to do anything special to clean.

Just take a bath and clean like normal. It's no big deal. I don't feel comfortable having this conversation.

My daughter taught me about douching.

Many years ago, I saw her filling a rubber bag with water. When I asked what it was, she said I should know. That hurt my feelings. She said it was a douche bag. Still a little hurt, I asked what's a douche bag. She said it's to clean the coochie. I asked her how. She explained and said it's something I should do regularly, and that she didn't believe I'd never done it. I hated that she talked to me like I was stupid. That's not something we learned when I was growing up.

The next day, she bought me one. Using it felt weird. You know, I don't even use tampons. But she had talked so much about how important it is for my health. So I did it. Eventually, I got used to it. Then last year, she changed her tune and went off that I shouldn't be doing that because it's bad for my health.

I was taught to start douching when I was 16.

But a few years back, my gynecologist said that women have the wrong idea about douching. She insisted that we shouldn't because a woman's period cleanses the impurities. Once I stopped having a period, I started douching again, but I don't encourage it to women who are still menstruating.

When I take a shower, I always spend a few extra moments on my the pubic hair.

I soap it down and scratch it real good. That's my way of making sure all of it—every strand of hair, every nook and cranny, is clean. I always have. No one taught me to do that. I just want to make sure it's real clean.

I grew up with that big, red rubber hot water bag hanging in the bathroom.

I know you know what I'm talking about. It was always saddling the shower curtain rod, with this long white nozzle beside it. When I asked my mom what it was, she said it was for tummy aches. When I got older, I realized it's also for douching. But to this day, my mom—who doesn't believe some things should be said out loud—still won't have a conversation about that secondary use.

From time to time, and I can't explain it, some women have an odor that hits you in a certain way. It is neither romantic nor encouraging. Instead, it elicits a reaction that makes it something I simply can't embrace. The smell is beyond pungent.

At that point, I can walk away or stay. There are two things that can create a bridge, allowing me to go on: I can turn my head a certain way, and maybe put a T-shirt over my nose and literally will myself to reconnect with my desire. Or, and this is a bit of a mind game, I can find a way to embrace the scent (See how I use the word scent instead of odor? It's all in the mind.) and to make it part of the enticement.

The way I see it,

a car isn't clean if you don't wash the tires; a house isn't clean if you don't do the windows; the bedroom isn't clean if you don't make the bed... and a woman's body isn't clean if she doesn't clean her bush. She needs to dig in and clean the vagina. Men too. Men need to move the ball sack around and really clean.

One night I was with this girl and I were about to have sex.

But she was really smelly down there. I didn't want to walk away from the moment, so I sprayed some perfume on it. Bad idea. The alcohol in the perfume reacted to her skin. Her pussy shriveled up and turned dark—like a bruise. It looked like someone had just punched her between the legs. She was burning. Her vagina was horrible to look at. Needless to say, we didn't have sex. But I felt I shouldn't leave, so I stayed with her the whole night.

In Cameroon, we use incense. Everyone has their own blend which can really vary among families and villages. It's very secretive. We don't tell anyone the ingredients. Being clean and having a beautiful scent is very important.

Whether she trims or shaves, has hair or doesn't, isn't important. Just as long as it's clean.

I went through a depression a while ago, and I forgot to really clean myself. Actually, I stopped doing a lot of things, but I can't believe I didn't do that either. It didn't even occur to me. Then at some point, every time I went to the bathroom, I smelled an odor and was like, "What is going on?" I thought my body was broken, which made me more depressed. I'm better now. Thank God.

I was living in the southern U.S. around the time women discovered Bath & Body Works. They all smelled like cucumber and pear. When it got hot, I could tell when it was that time for some women to "freshen up" because they had the whole mall smelling like a rancid fruit salad.

The first time I douched, I liked it.

I'd always wanted a fresh flower scent. I don't know why I wanted my coochie to smell like a daisy. I think it might be because of the white lady on the box running through the field of flowers. She looked so happy.

I stopped when my doctor told me it wasn't good for me and that that's why I was getting yeast infections. When I stopped, I didn't get anymore infections.

Clean your face, your ears, your belly button, your ass and your dick.

Sometimes I think motherfuckers might forget about their feet, might forget about their elbows, might forget about their neck—but you not gonna forget about the most important parts. You not gon' forget to clean under your arms, clean your dick.

My friend douches all the time and she still stinks.

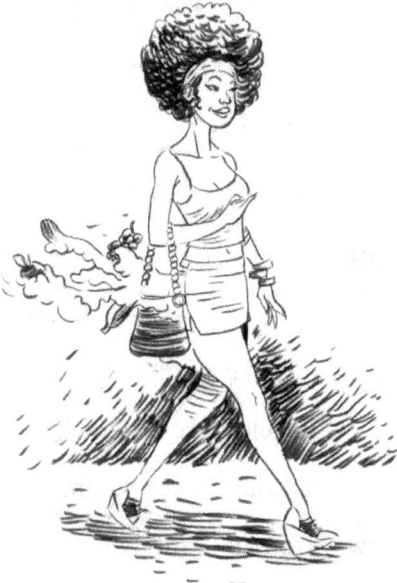

Moerat Sitompul

You take a stick of Degree deodorant

(Fresh Shower Scent) and wipe it on your upper thigh, along the edge of the pantyline—back and forth, right there in that leg crease. It takes away the wetness in your panties and keeps you smelling fresh all day. And every now and then, swipe it up your ass. Because that's where hair grows and your ass will smell fresh. Not a lot. Just a little swipe that's all you need. I don't do it everyday in the ass, but definitely in the front, near the man-trap.

I'll say something like, maybe you need to take a shower.

Sometimes, I get nervous if someone bends down to pick up something near my waist. Even though I shower and stay clean, I'm still afraid they might be hit with an odor. So when they bend down, I usually take a step back, or offer to help so I can bend down too. Anything to keep them away from my pantyline. It's a phobia.

I like the pubic hair. It traps the scent, and I like the scent.

A woman can do anything. She can literally stab a man, but if she's got that sex smell, he's not going anywhere. He will still be with her. That smell is a smell a guy needs. All mammals are drawn to smell. You've gotta have it. If you don't, there's no attraction.

Growing up in Colombia, I just remember being a little girl and putting a bar of soap inside of me when I was taking a bath. It burned so bad that I just always had this image that soap is bad for you down there.

If you keep it clean, it shouldn't matter if you have hair or not.

In Sweden, we're pretty open about personal hygiene.

My mom was so excited when I started my period that she called and told both of my aunts and my grandmother. She explained how sometimes I'll want to freshen up, then took me to the bathroom and showed me how to use the removable showerhead to properly clean myself. I remember she had me take off my pants and underwear, and stand in the tub. Then she literally climbed into the tub with me and showed me how I have to lift one leg up and rest it on the edge of the tub, and turn the showerhead upside down to properly wash myself.

There's a fetish for dick cheese,

the white crust that builds up if you haven't washed after sex (or at all) for a long time. It's called smegma, and men and women both get it if they're not clean. It's thick enough that you can take a spoon, scrape it off, and spread it on toast. I think that's the height of poor hygiene.

Don't tell anyone this, but I sometimes eat naked.

And when I drop food, I pick the crumbs out of my crotch and eat them. I'm just saying, that's how clean I keep things down there.

I was living in the U.S. for years before I heard of douches.

In Japan, I'd never heard of products like that. Odor is not a problem. Maybe it's because we regularly bathe in the onsen. Or maybe it's our diet, but Japanese people don't have an odor. It's never a problem.

In Ghana, we douche with clove-infused water after our periods.

Clove water is really good for women. We sometimes use it to wash outside of the vulva, between our legs, whenever we want to feel fresh, and we sit over a steam bath of cloves and hot water after giving birth to help our vaginal canal heal more quickly.

In the Caribbean, we're taught to wash our underwear when we take a shower.

We throw our other clothes in the washing machine, but we handwash our underwear while we're taking shower. Then hang them on hooks to dry. It's considered hygienic. For us, it's natural, but my dad, who's American, hates it. He thinks it's embarrassing for guests to use the bathroom and see underwear hanging. But what they do is better? Leaving their underwear in a pile of clothes to just sit in their juices?

In Niger, as a Muslim, we're taught to thoroughly wash our privates after using the bathroom. (Not just dry-wiping with toilet tissue.) Living abroad, many Muslims won't use the bathroom at their jobs or in public places because we don't like to just wipe. Personally, I keep my cup with me. I call it my cooch cup. After I finish using the bathroom, I get out my cup.

I was a dorm parent at a boarding school and issues like this came up all the time. Someone different came to me with a complaint every week, usually about hygiene. We had a lot of international students and everyone had different customs. And I'm not their parent. I didn't know what to say. And sometimes the other girls could be really mean.

I'm Guinean. Even though I was born in the U.S., I have always washed my drawers when I take a shower. I assumed everyone from the Diaspora did. When I go to Guinea, everyone does it. When I was in Nigeria, they did it. In Benin, they did it. When I traveled to the Caribbean, they did it. I was surprised that Black Americans don't. I had a Puerto Rican roommate who didn't. She asked, "Aren't you worried about getting it clean?" I said, "No. I'm more worried about just dropping it in a clothes basket, and leaving it to mix in with the rest of my laundry."

There's no shame in it. You just shower, wash your drawers, and hang them on the curtain rod. But since I have roommates who don't do that, I use a drying rack in my room. I'm very open about it.

In Russia when I was growing up, we didn't have tampons and sanitary pads.

We had to go to the pharmacy and stock up on cotton balls and gauze. We used something like a rubber harness that we tied around our panties and waist to hold everything in place.

This was still in the days of the Soviet Union. I lived in St. Petersburg. In my apartment, we had a bathtub in our kitchen. It was a huge kitchen, and the bathtub was there. A lot of apartments didn't even have that. People would go once a week to a *banya*—a public steam room. Back then, I was not on top of my hygiene. I was not taking good care of myself. I definitely was not taking a shower everyday. I think the ritual was once a week.

But we washed our privates every night before going to bed. We were taught to do that on the toilet with a jar of water. We would fill a jar with boiled water, go in the bathroom, sit on the toilet, and wash ourselves.

We have a bidet at home. My sons are so used to it that they won't even use public bathrooms. When they're at school, they just hold it until they come home.

In Korea, we generally live with our parents until we get married. The only thing my mom ever told me to keep clean was my room. And to not get my clothes dirty. Beyond just telling me to take a shower, we never had conversations about intimate hygiene. We learn some of it in high school, but they don't go into that much detail. I guess we pretty much learn on our own.

Like my mom says, "Ain't no man gone want you with dirty underwear."

When I see women wearing short skirts on the subway I cringe.

The look is cute when they're standing up. But when they sit down, there is nothing to protect them from all of the dirt, sweat, fart gas and billions of germs and bacteria on the seats. They're laughing and talking, not even realizing how dirty they are.

In China, public bathrooms don't have doors on the stalls. I don't see how you can maintain good hygiene when you don't even have basic privacy.

A friend posted on Facebook once that she tried those period panties. She said they were the worst things ever. I didn't understand how she thought they'd be anything but a disaster.

When I take a dump, I wipe two times. That's it. If there's still anything up in there after that, it's just gonna have to stay until the next time.

Public bathrooms are common in Korea and many of them have bidets. Whenever I go to the toilet and see a bidet, I'm like "Wooo!" Men don't really think about cleanliness in the same way women do, but I really like bidets.

How can you be in somebody's face,

talking and kissing, and you stink. What's up with that?

My system shuts down. When there's

somebody that needs to be cleaned, my system shuts down and I can't reboot myself. I don't conscientiously choose to shut down. It just happens. And don't let it be there first time I've met you.

I still remember my mom saying, "You stink. I need to teach you how to wash your ass because you stink." She took me in the shower, got in there with me and showed me how to properly clean in between my butt cheeks. I mean, this happened when I was a kid. I was like, three, at the time. But I still remember it. She just kept saying that I stink.

If it's sexual, there are pheremones that... you know what I mean, will wake you up. It makes me bring on the heat. There's heat going on with certain odors. When the heat is there, that's a whole other thing. But when it's something else—when you have not washed your ass and there's bacteria making you stink, I can't be around you.

You have to wipe until it comes out clean.

Men:

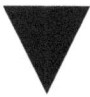

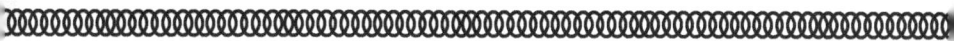

Shaving & manscaping

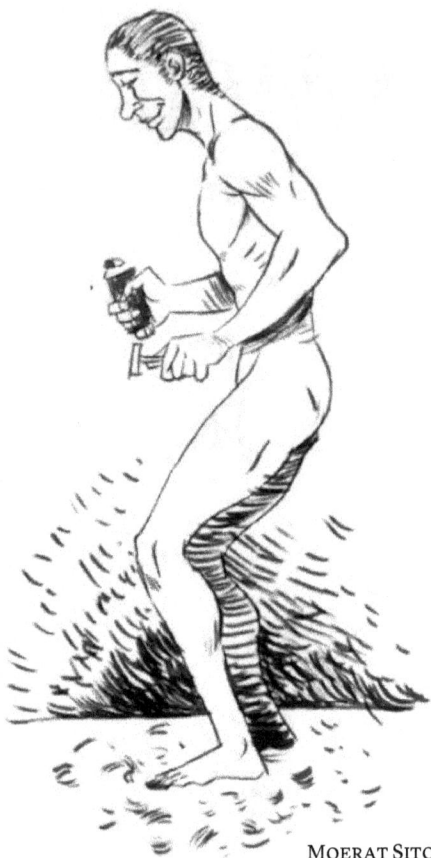

MOERAT SITOMPUL

We can't just let that shit grow long. It's not about the smell. As men, we're gonna have an odor either way. But it gets sweaty down there, and sweat stinks.

Some men shave all the hair off. It's one thing to shave the balls, but everything?

It makes them look like a man-child, like a baby. I noticed that it's common among Dominican men, and some Black men. I don't know if it's a comfort thing. Personally, I like it trimmed instead of completely shaven.

Shaving the balls is more common with us white guys because we tend to get pretty hairy. And it gets long and straggly. Personally, I shave regularly for cycling. The less I have down there, the better. If I don't, I chafe.

San Francisco is like the leather bear capital of the world. In Los Angeles, I can see men following that trend and shaving down there. But in San Francisco, men are hairy like bears.

I "Nair" my butt hole. I use the hell

out of a depilatory—I put it on everything, down to my ankles. When I'm rubbing it on my butt, I'm like, "Fuck it," and put it in the hole, too. I don't like a hairy butt. It makes it sweat and smell more.

We have to be very careful. I use

a regular razor, but I take my time. We don't want to be in a hurry—don't want to nick something. That is very painful.

Hahahahaha!

I have the same hair on my dick that I've had since I was ten. It hasn't changed. Men don't shave, baby. Hear me? MEN don't shave.

I hate guys who think they're too manly to trim. That shit gets nappy.

Anal hair is— forgive the pun—a pain in the ass. The only way to really get at it is by waxing. I guess that or using a depilatory. One of the many reasons I'm not homosexual is my aversion for hair. I don't like body hair. I go through very specific times when I shave down there and I can be very pedantic about it.

I used to care what other people thought about me shaving, but as I've gotten older, I care less and less about other people's opinions.

Because it's nappy? No, uh, uh. If it's nappy, curly, long, straight, whatever. That's the way it's supposed to be.

Stink? That's what it's supposed to do. That's what showers were made for.

I thought it was cool when I first got pubic hair.

I thought I was grown. When I first felt hair on my dick, I was like, wow! Me and my cousin talked about it. It was one of those things—a sign of maturity. "I got something on my nuts! Now let's get some more."

I was shy the first time I shaved and tapered. So much so, that I stopped calling my girlfriend. I just

didn't think she'd accept it. Later on, she saw me in the laundromat

and asked why I had stopped calling. I told her. I remember that I

was wearing shorts at the time, and sitting on one of the machines.

She came in close and rubbed my legs. "Hmmm, smooth," she said.

She asked how much I shaved off. I told her all of it. She asked

if she could feel it. I said yeah. We worked things out over the spin

cycle, so to speak.

What do you call your penis?

Cock Dong

Lizard

JOHNSON

Schlong WAND

snake

Schwantz
(German for tail)

God's Gift

MANHOOD NUTS

Twig and Cherry

Mini-Me DRIBBLER

One-Eyed Wonder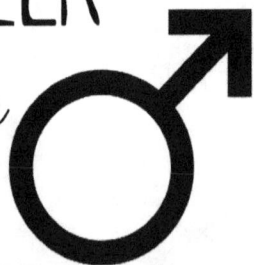

DINGALING

I've never even seen shaving instruments for men. What do they use?

Certainly not the same razor that they use on their face?

I don't shave. I like it hairy. I think

there are a lot of men—gay and straight—who don't like it smooth. I mean, if you're naturally smooth, that's fine. But if you shave, then you're unnaturally smooth. That's kind of feminine.

I didn't pay any attention to mine and then one day, I just started. I don't even remember that first time, except for the fact that it was after my divorce. It was sort of revelatory. I thought, "Huh, I could cut this." It just seemed like the thing to do. "Neaten it up a little bit, get it out of the way a little bit." I was single. I did it for myself. That was in 1986. I liked it and I still do it.

Manscaping is nice. Guys should trim it down so that it's nice to look at.

I guess what can be done with hair and how it's approached can be fun.

Back in Miami, as a professional swimmer, I trained, lifted, and body-sculpted a lot. I made an offhanded complaint to one of my female friends one day about how I have to shave but didn't feel like it. She offered to do it for me. We were at her place. She spread a blanket on the floor in the living room. She lathered me down and started shaving. There wasn't that much, so it was more of a touch-up. Her roommate came home with a friend, and it became a party. It grew into a regular thing. I was their toy.

I don't know if this is throughout South Korea, but my uncle taught me an important lesson. One day I was complaining that the hair around my penis itched. He told me that when I take a shower, I should always rinse it with conditioner. I thought he was nuts, but the next day, I tried it. It worked.

It's not like I go around talking about this stuff with other guys, but I have mentioned it a couple of times. And then they tried it and came back to me and said the same thing. It really works.

Trimming helps my stroke. Most men don't

know their sexual stroke number, but I've paid attention. The first
time I shaved, I noticed I lasted longer having sex. And I shoot
further. My orgasm is stronger. When you get older, every stroke
matters.

I shave for women. It's not for me. As more women are getting rid of their bush, I think men need to put in some effort and meet them halfway. I don't shave everything and I don't do it all the time. But I do try to be mindful that sometimes that shit might be uncomfortable for them.

I can't say I'm opposed to the idea, or in favor of it. I just think guys who shave have a lot of extra time on their hands. I work for a living. And when I get home, I want a beer. Not a razor so I can cut the hair around my dick.

Men:

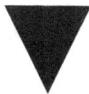

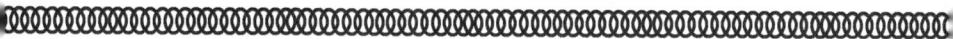

What women say

Some men can have peasy hair. I didn't really like it but I thought I had to deal with it because of the notion that "real men" don't groom. As soon as I realized that men can and do shave their scrotal hair, I decided to talk to my boyfriend about it. He thought I was out of my mind and I never brought it up again. Later on, after we broke up, I started dating a guy who happened to trim. It was nice. I looked at him differently—in a good way—like, he was man enough to do something like that and not question his manhood.

I don't care if he doesn't shave. I like

a little hair. Not a mouthful though. Before I get a mouthful of hair, I would prefer that he at least trim.

I've seen men with pubic hair longer than their penises. Their dicks look

like garden gnomes. Like a little hat popping out from the grass. It's especially funny looking if he's uncircumcised.

Guys need to learn to trim if they want somebody to suck on it, especially if they just shake it off all day after using the bathroom, instead of wiping with tissue. No, if it's not trimmed, it's not happening.

I'm dating a guy who shaves it all off. The first time I saw it, I thought it was a little weird. But I'm used to it now. Actually, I guess now I like it better because if he let his hair grow, it'll be gray and I think that might turn me off.

These guys running around dating younger women... I know they must be dyeing down there.

When I was 22, I dated a 40-year-old. He was such a ladies' man, and so proud to be dating this young woman. We broke up and went our separate ways for awhile. One night while we were talking about getting back together, he mentioned gray hair as a hypothetical, and I just freaked. I was like, "Eww!! That's disgusting. I don't ever want to see that!" He got silent and just clammed up. I realized he must have been talking about himself. Maybe he had been gray all along and got tired of dyeing it, or maybe it was a new development. But in any case, I imagine he went out and stocked up his supply of Clairol the next day.

I think men shave because they think it'll make their thing look bigger than it really is. I think a lot of guys are smaller than they want to be or think they should be. They're all about "I want to maximize how I look." I don't think they're thinking about hygiene at all.

I look at his hair and his eyebrows. If I see he's bald, I just assume he's pretty hairless down there too. And then I discover, "Wow, you're holding out!"

Many thanks to everyone who supported *Down There*: Baden Copeland for the original cover design, Monica Williams for proofreading, and Jen Spence, Moerat Sitompul and Veronica Malatesta for their amazing illustrations, ...

... and to everyone who contributed their stories. Because I promised that your contributions would be anonymous, I cannot thank you by name. But you know who are.

Treadwater • Breathe Publishing

DOWN THERE

Georgia Scott is a visual communicator and internationalist. Seeking out grassroots projects that explore the sameness of humankind, she has traveled to 69 countries and taught or conducted workshops in seven, including as a Knight Fellow in Indonesia and China; a visiting professional with U.S. Embassies in Burma and South Korea, and as a freelancer in Peru for the United Nations. Georgia worked in the editorial art department at *The New York Times* for 15 years, owned an international coffeehouse and bookstore in Harlem, and taught journalism and editorial design at universities in New York and Hawaii. Currently, she works at an NGO in South Korea, where she also teaches business and conversation English.

Other titles by Georgia Scott:
Headwraps: A Global Journey (2003, Public Affairs)
How Langston Leaf Delayed Winter (2010, Treadwater-Breathe)
Everyday Hugs (2011, Treadwater-Breathe)
Good Hugs, Bad Hugs (2011, Treadwater-Breathe)
Worth the Wait (2015, Treadwater-Breathe)

Treadwater Breathe is an international, creative storyhouse that promotes dialogue, original content, and the successful start of difficult conversations.

To join the discussion:

Down There is an authentic tool for men and women around the world to begin openly discussing their interest, or lack thereof, of intimate grooming and hygiene. To publicly join the discussion, and possibly be included in the next edition, please visit: www.iamgeorgiascott.com